Physically Deteriorating, Emotionally Distressing

Who I Am With FA

Yesenia Ramos

ISBN-13: 9781798430446

Yesenia Ramos

CONTENTS

Acknowledgement i

Poem I   Weep in Silence
Poem II   Crybaby Throne
Poem III   Within a Non-Refundable Body
Poem IV   Helpful possession
Poem V   Night-Time Struggles
Poem VI   Oh, Grief
Poem VII   Yells Anxiety
Poem VIII   All Dysarthria
Poem IX   Tired of being Fatigued
Poem X   "If you're Living, then you're Dying"
Poem XI   Cure FA
Poem XII   I'm Here
Poem XIII   Please, Don't Say I Can't Handle Anything
Poem XIV   God Have Mercy
Poem XV   Harder and Harder
Poem XVI   Faith?
Poem XVII   Unanswered Questions
Poem XVIII   Nothing Ever Happens
Poem XIX   Hate
Poem XX   Lost Me
Poem XXI   What Am I?
Poem XXII   Ingredients of Myself
Poem XXIII   Self-Religious
Poem XXIV   Ask The Shamans
Poem XV   From The Beginning
Poem XXVI   Also Known As FA
Poem XXVII   Interesting to Look At
Poem XXVIII   Hidden Hearing Loss
Poem XXIX   With This Progression, i Survive
Poem XXX   Homebound til further Notice
Poem XXXI   FAmily

ACKNOWLEDGMENTS

I would like to dedicate my first poetic project; so abysmal and full of emotions, to a dear friend named Ronald Salugao. We met in a depression/anxiety support group; he observed that I needed a healthy coping mechanism. He introduced me to poetry all this is happening because of him! Also, I want to dedicate this book to my 3 cousins, Nayeli Talamantes, Elizabeth Ramos and Daniel Torres. They're my rock, my supporters, my #1 fans, I wouldn't be putting myself out there if it wasn't for there love and motivation.🙏🤍

Weep in Silence

I have this monster in my head
growling, causing a migraine
I just clinch my jaw hard
telling myself that the deafening, painful, howls will stop
soon enough
but what am I supposed to do now since the monster
found its way through my nerves
my blood is scorching
it's unbearable
this horrendous parasite wants me to react
I tighten up my fists and let this anger agitate me inside
out
even my tears are sizzling
my thoughts are building up
they're making everything worse
bloody lava is oozing out my skull
I prefer this frustration, self-hatred, fury. only abuse me
I'm not one to share my pain
I'm one to put everyone first
and i know that letting people all the way in will turn into
many heartbreaks
so tears stream down my face as I cover my mouth and
weep in silence

Crybaby Throne

I'm not sensitive
I'm hypersensitive
I sometimes wish for a sedative
I'm effortlessly hurt
I'm lightly worried
I'm uncomplicatedly offended
saying 'NO' to someone makes me feel downhearted
I'm sadly unsettled
but I keep my emotions safely bottled
being yelled at belittles my pride and ego
sometimes I'm in need of a superhero
although my vulnerability stays unknown
I sit in a crybaby throne
"get rid of your dogs, your parents can't take care of you,
your brother and your 2 dogs"
just pause for a second, imagine how I feel hearing that
impotence, weary-load, helplessness
stating comments that compare me to my brother
emerges this great fear inside me
"will my disability progress that much too?"
"will I be as cruel as he is to my parents?"
"is that part of our disability?"
"does god want me to turn out like my brother?"
"is god trying to teach my parents a lesson?"
"what if god makes my fear come true?"
faith never turns out good for me
with that being said I'm not having it
I'm ultra-sensible to pain
I have a right to be afraid of change, the future, even
sometimes the present
I'm in a oversensitive emotional state

Within a Non-Refundable Body

I didn't ask for a body that doesn't work
but I got one
one, that makes me want to point a gun to my temple
one, infested with Friedreichs Ataxia
a body God created
yet people say it's not his fault
it's tremendously prejudiced
seeing other people enjoy life yet not being able to enjoy it
myself
I have stayed up many nights questioning "why couldn't I
have a body like everyone else's"
I never get an answer
my body is too delicate
it malfunctions too much
many times, I've desired to return my body
If only reincarnation was a sure thing
this body makes me scream and cry
I want to know what god was thinking
did he know i was going to go through hell emotionally
did he think I deserved this life
I have days I even wish I was never born
so I wouldn't have this broken body
I doubt god is as good as everyone says
he has the power to fix me but doesn't
it's harsh, cruel and distressing
I'm better off not believing
I've grown to fear him
within a nonrefundable, Friedreichs Ataxian body

Helpful Possession

do you know what it feel like to be like this

to be betrayed by your own body

to wonder with terror if you'll be alive next year or in 2 years

to hurt more than you can effectively express

to want to do something you know you can't physically bring to a successful conclusion

to be haunted by the next limitation due to the progression

the intimidation, the feebleness, the helplessness I must feel

my body is in chaos

big reason why I go through depression

mourning is part of the procession

I have tried therapy sessions

but I've found poetry is my only helpful possession

Night-Time Struggles

does any of you have to think about turning sides at night

how many of you think about moving your legs when you're half asleep

none, right

most people at night moan because they're having sex

I moan due to the strength it takes to simply turn sides in my bed

sometimes, I sound like I'm fighting a t-rex

it's hardwork

I even sweat and I have to pause to catch my breath as if I was doing fieldwork

it's tough for FA to let me rest

if I'm not laying on my pillow right, my muscles get tense

it gets intense

imagine having to wake up at 3AM to massage your own neck

to try to relieve the pain in your muscles

too sleep like a baby, I need miracles

night time is as long as tunnels

but the length isn't good

I'm awake half the time with these FA troubles

that's just my night-time struggles

Oh, Grief

losing loved ones is my possible weakness

a life changing event that's so grievous

the heaviness is life altering

it's suffering, languishing, lamenting 24/7

with fidgety nights, full of nightmares

it's a time of sadness where I need empathy and sympathy

a time you'd like to experience no more than once

I find myself stuck dreading the next time

it's a great heartache I try to dodge

but it's inescapable morosely

cancer is the most wanted serial killer

then comes Alzheimer's

then car accidents

I wish the deploring didn't leave wounds jkj

I won't lie, sometimes I ask for the despair to be physical torture

I am even careful on how close I get to people

that's how traumatized I am

oh, grief!

I guess if you want love, you have to be prepared to go through the pain

Yells Anxiety

.

Uncoordinated movements

it's being drunk while In a state of sobriety

clumsiness is a big cause of my anxiety

worrying about grabbing, touching, moving, holding, reaching for, and placing objects

every abnormal thing comes with stares in our society

which Yells ANXIETY

fearing my disability and the unaccepting community

unusual awkwardness moving arms, legs, hands, feet, fingers

I'm presumably different

different equals weird and weird yells ANXIETY

All Dysarthria

"what?" "can you repeat that?" "I can't understand you"

my sounds run into one another

it's a bother

I say I speak cursive

not gorgeous calligraphic swirls

more like 2nd grade cursive

I mumble, stammer, garble

have you been drinking?

well, I think physically my body is intoxicated

but mentally I'm one hundred percent non-indulgent

my mind is in order

I'm not fond of repeating myself

I think twice before saying anything

I'm insecure of my speech

it's all Dysarthria

Tired of being Fatigued

fatigue

Unrelenting exhaustion

of course it's a symptom of FA

I hate it

it makes me want to quit

it leaves me without motivation and concentration

my life's full of frustration

I wish I could fix fatigue with medication

not even coffee gives me that bit of energy I need

just makes my heart skip a beat

being sleepy is not even close to fatigue

you don't comprehend the annoyance

the lingering tiredness is consuming

it's constant and limiting

you get tired of being fatigued

"If You're Living, then You're Dying"

FA can kill you

google it, it's so true

it is depressing

it's what has me nervous, paranoid and stressing

it's why I fear the future, truly dreadful

I'm scared of death in general

it affects my mental

cardiomyopathy is what kills everyone with FA, regretfully

If not heart failure

I live with that expectancy

I wish I could change that

I wish it wasn't fatal

but "if you're living, you're dying " that goes for everyone

Cure FA

There is a piece inside
the void
the grief
there is so much damage
and change that it is haunting
it's like my body is possessed
I'm not the woman I wanted to be
how disappointing
This woman turned out to be different
not the woman my mom or my dad hoped I'd be
I can't help but ask myself if people, my family, are
ashamed of me
I'm the woman who's nerves connect abnormally
so my muscles don't react normally
But my heart can feel
and the loss of my abilities surreal
Will a cure for FA ever come?

I'm Here

when I say I'm here, then I'm here
I mean it
I'm here honestly, sometimes painfully so
perhaps I don't have firsthand experience with the exact
thing you're going through
but I know what it means to hurt
Hurt translates pretty well
I know what it's like to be in a room full of people but
feeling alone
I know what it's like to be so desperate for the emotional
damage to be turned off
you hurt yourself to distract yourself
I know what it's like to feel like even talking about it is
nothing but a pointless stirring of air
I care too much for any soul to feel that way alone
so I'm here
I'd give you my time, my love, my arms & ears
And don't you worry because I won't butt in
I'll let you speak to your heart's content
I'm here if you need a shoulder to cry on
wet my shirt with your tears
sob all you want
I won't judge you
i know I can't take your hurting away
but I can be by your side while you fix yourself
I know what it's like and I don't want anyone to endure it
too
sadly, I recognize it's ineluctable
but what isn't is letting you walk through hell alone
I'm here

Please, Don't say I Can't Handle Anything

YoU CaNt HaNdLe AnYtHiNg
try being diagnosed with Friedreich's Ataxia at age 5
and your first memory being of your mom bawling at the doctors office
try being in 5th grade and warning your friends that you'll be crippled in 6th grade
popularity and friendships are valued a lot during that time
but, try seeing everyone start treating you different
due to something you can't control
try going from popular to outcast
something like that sticks with you

I'm not done yet though
try having your first boyfriend ever tell you how gross you are to him
try being asked over and over again "what happened to you?"
and answering that you fell down stairs
for, the real reason you're ashamed of
try crying "I want my mom" with the anesthesia already being inhaled
try being forced to stand up after surpassing a surgery
try thinking you'd rather die than recover
only for the physical pain to stop

try having in mind "What if you never recover" "this is too hard, it's unfair" "you'll probably recover but nothing will be the same" every single second
try making a teacher give up on you
as a justification to not get extra help
to feel independent
try getting 28 detentions
the reason being for acting disrespectful, the bad kind of defensive, rude
try seeing a teacher like a second mom
And getting extremely, dangerously attached
try having a explosive school year
where you got suspended and expelled in the same week
try being told your school mom quit
try not knowing what to do, so you just sit in the restroom skipping every class
With every other teacher belittling your emotions, feeling alone and like a joke
try dropping out the first day of senior year
it being so overwhelming you couldn't go back

I really wish I was done but not quite

try being misunderstood, misinterpreted for carrying your heart on your sleeve
try wanting to talk to someone who doesn't want to talk to you
try hitting your head so much you're scared that the next time might be the last time
Try losing your grandpa in 2016 and your baby cousin in 2017
All in Mexico
try going to Mexico to visit they're resting place but being to terrified to get out of bed

try being emotionally and verbally abused by your older brother
try seeing your brother call the police on your mom
and when a officer talks to you, you literally freeze and sob
try witnessing your brother hit your parents
try knowing to call the police but being too afraid to

still think I can't handle anything?

God Have Mercy

GOD you woke up from the dead
you resuscitated
Why do I have to be wheelchair bound
Why do I have to have the disease Friedreich's Ataxia
Is there a lesson I should be learning
Can you not cure me
my life's a suffering spree
depression and anxiety attack me
Friedreich's Ataxia kills me slowly, literally
      GOD HAVE MERCY
I don't want to hear that it is not in your power
theirs been cases where people get miraculously cured
explain yourself
Is it that you just hate me
Am I undeserving
      GOD PLEASE HAVE MERCY
tell me, how do you want me to start believing you're good
if you won't even do this little thing for me
I need to be saved, can you not see that

Harder and Harder

I always try my best
but I'm way too good at faking it when stressed
it's hard, scary as fuck to say you're depressed
my emotions could be spurned
or plain out refused to be acknowledged
truth is, it wears me out
seeing everyone around me happy is crappy
my family, cousins, friends
makes me feel lonesome and melancholy
for, I find myself contemplating suicide with a jolly outer
layer
the thing is I don't want to die
I don't want to leave my loved ones
I'm a really selfless person
but I need my pain to stop
give me another solution to remove my emotional
soreness
because I don't want to ask for help
I've gone there, I done that
it's not for me
you're forced to open up to a complete strangers
I'm not a fan
just fill me up with Zoloft, Prozac, Lexapro
simply multiply my milligrams
for, faking it is getting harder and harder

Faith?

it has been 156 years since FA was discovered

I have suffered 16 long-lasting years

how am I supposed to still have faith?

it's as hard as believing in something you can't see

if I doubt God, then I'll obviously doubt for a cure to be found while I'm living

sounds pessimistic but I'm only stating how I think

try dealing with depression/anxiety and staying optimistic

my thoughts are realistic

but most people can't bare with my realism

people enjoy the inspiration porn

that's today's generation

Nicholaus Friedreich wouldn't be proud of our progression

Unanswered Questions

will I ever get to walk again before I die?

why doesn't my oldest brother not really talk to me?

is this disease some sort of punishment from God?

is God good or bad?

does it make me a bad person if I choose to be non-religious because I'm mad at God?

if I do something disrespectful, rude or spiteful will God punish me?

what does God think?

are people right, am I too much to handle?

does my disability make me ugly?

who'll be the next person in my life to pass away?

should I feel bad because some people have it worse?

do my parents suffer because I'm hurting?

am I worthy of love?

how am I seen in people's eyes?

these are my unanswered questions

I'm afraid of some of the answers

Nothing Ever Happens

I didn't wanna awake my mom to help me at night

so I cried frustratedly loud

like a baby

I couldn't end my tears

"what do I do now?" "please God do something!"

I could feel the empathy in the air

I just felt my moms heart break while hearing her daughter in frustration and desperation

I kept telling myself to stop but I just couldn't

I looked up with tears streaming down face, whispering "help me"

I have days I'm so desperate I beg God

but nothing ever happens

Hate

I hate the words
   I'm
     sorry
       you
        have
          Friedreich's Ataxia
I hate the metal rods in my back area
I hate feeling emotionally trapped, anxious about the future and the inability to protect
I hate how my senses decrease due to the FA effect
I hate the inability to walk, coordinate, balance, have 20/20 vision
I hate the fatigueness, people call fiction
I hate the albeism and discrimination
I hate my heart condition which makes my life shorten
I hate spasms and spasticity
I hate receiving pity
I hate the finger triggers
especially when I stretch my fingers
I hate taking medicine, day and night
I hate that I cannot normally function
I hate judgements, adjustments and modifications
Everywhere transitions
I hate accommodations
I hate when people are stereotypical
I hate choking on nothing but air and saliva
it leaves me coughing and gasping like I'm being strangled
prisoned in restless rest until FA decides it is done with me

I hate the deformities of my feet
I hate surgeries
I hate being dependent
I hate that the messages coming from my Cerebellum can't always reach the body parts I want to move
I hate my disability that I feel screams out 'she's defective'
I hate handicapped stickers
I hate being physically and emotionally broken
I hate being betrayed by my disloyal body
I hate the uncertainty, the inability to plan for the future
I hate having to acknowledge that I have FA out loud
I hate Friedreich's Ataxia
But
I love life
guess it all evens out
Guess I'm more okay than not

Lost Me

life was barely commencing
at age 6, it was the beginning
I was full of innocence
my hardest problem was subtraction
along came Friedreich's Ataxia
it is my diagnosis, Dr.'s say
my life plan was rearranged
I wish my fate was exchanged
at age 6 everything changed
at age 6 I defined the words pity and stressed
FA abruptly stole my ability and independence
at age 6 I lost me
my faith was supposed to keep me afloat but I lost that too

Fear of rejection, depression and anxiety
Obstacles, there are so many
I can't find me

Attitude, they say, stay positive
Cure?
there is none
Surely they'll find one
Uncertainty?
There is plenty
I'm broken emotionally
I guess physically too
I've been lost for a long period
I'm no longer six, amber alerts don't exist
I'm only found when I reminisce

more progressed, more profoundly I go to the bottomless abyss
Eradicate FA, and guide me back

What am I?

I am from both of your parents

I decide which nervous system to affect greatly

it's all about luck

I am linked to the gene FXN

a gene I lack

I am intelligent, degenerative & progressive

I incapacitate my prey at various levels

I am different with everybody

I develop impaired muscle coordination that worsens over time

oftentimes I create heart disease

and cause gradual loss of strength, sensation in the arms and legs, muscle stiffness, impaired speech, hearing, and vision

my addiction is putting my targets out of commission

what am I?

Ingredients to Myself

in a baking pan add Friedreichs Ataxia

cover with mental illness cream (depression and anxiety)

2 pounds of frustration cut into 2 inch cubes

then add 3 tablespoons of humor oil

Include 4 bone-in of fake smiles chops

3/4 cups of emotional distress

Also a 1/2 cup of bashfulness combined with the same amount of fear

1 teaspoon of volunteer work

Mix in a pinch of attitude

cook for 30-45 minutes

Sprinkle some art and advertising talents at the end

And you have made a replica of me!

Self-Religious

Catholic?

Christianity?

Hinduism?

Islam?

Buddhism?

What am I?

I guess I'm a broken religion

I'm not sure of anything

If God is as pleasant as everyone expresses, then why would he give me this hella life?

What did I do to condign this?

It's injustice

How do you 'God' expect me to live?

I never receive my remarkably needed responses

Is anyone up there?

Can you hear my plea for help?

Are you discrediting my yell?

Am I invisible?

Not even a megaphone works to be seen or heard

Suicide is in my head and you're neglecting my shouts for assistance

I'm beginning to think no one's up there

Ask the Shamans

shaman, religious specialist, curer, nonmedical therapist, or mender

whatever you know them by

I've seen a total of five

five faith healers

at first, I didn't know whether to believe these alternative practitioners

my beliefs became such flusters

at age six my religion was broken but I didn't know

true desperation brings you to believe in the unknown

as seen on TV

a unique, profound, desperation

I believe, only parents of disableds feel

divine healings do happen as seen as TV

it's a reason why I stay up asking God "why not grant me the miracle?" "do you think I don't deserve one?"

where do you think my anger towards God comes from?

why does he heal others and not me?

these faith healers made me puzzled, bewildered, & doubtful

if you wonder where my faith stands

ASK THE SHAMANS

instead of making my life easy, they made it questionable

From the Beginning

we have the same disease, permanently
Friedrelch's Ataxia is heredity
it's like a life penalty
scientifically, medically, biologically, genetically
that doesn't mean, the things that happen to your life is
going to happen in mine
that's a big false
it's a psychological decline
we might be physically equal
but our soul differs completely
stop making me believe otherwise
you pull my strings constantly
being compared to you is carelessly depressing
You cause more stressing than blessings
by opening your huge mouth your traumatizing
obviously you don't see it or you don't care
this has been happening from the beginning
ever since I received my diagnosis
I actually came to think FA was contagious
I blame your heinous and traumatic comments
you took advantage of my vulnerable moments
what a childhood I lived
and your abuse has worsened
it carrys on
i'm just holding in my reactions
"if you have nothing nice to say, don't say nothing at all"
but at this point, it's not healthy
when I blow up I'm going to end up like the bad person,
resenting
even though I'll only be defending

34

Also known as FA

Loss of coordination
loss of proprioception
surgical interventions
vision/hearing impairment
jerky eye movements
Muscle weakness
emotional distress
absent deep tendon reflexes
scoliosis
High plantar arches
slurred speech
heart disorder
dependency
balance difficulty
spasticity
wheelchair bound
extreme fatigue
suffering daily
slowly progressing

Interesting to Look At

when you're in a wheelchair people stare

they look at you from top to bottom

and when your feet are mildly deformed

well, that just makes me more interesting to look at

miffed, irked, disgruntled

I have sensitive feet

when my mom puts my socks on, it's like hot stabbing knives in the soles of my feet

my bottom half of myself exasperates me so much I want to cut it off

shoes are now almost impossible to put on and I'm a girl, so shoes are importance

surgery only repaired one of my feet

the other only got worse

recently, I've seen both of my feet getting really bad again

it so sad

I told myself no more surgeries

Hidden Hearing Loss

it's quite disheartening

not hearing in groups

only one on one

also known as hidden hearing loss

when this happens I can feel the judgments

"is she that disoriented?"

it's humiliating asking for repetition

society makes it all a saddening situation

distraught, shamefaced, agitated

I have this instinct that people began to associate my
hearing loss with my disability being mental

this results in getting sentimental

I can't help but be ashamed

I'll be honest it damages my self esteem

but maybe it's just me, my hesitancies

on the other hand it's erratic to think it's all facts

With this Progression, I Survive

I never liked wearing glasses

they are transforming

something I'm not a fan of

you see, I've always feared being bullied

my outcome being, never wearing my lenses in public

I avoided my fear, my great profession

as my disability is, my vision progressed

I failed my vision test

my eyesight changed and I had too change with it

the need of glasses triggered my apprehension towards adaptation

change is my agitation

wistfully, I hate it

I've grown to dismay life transitioning

i have PTSD in results of altering

my disability defines progression

equal to adjusting

the core to my depression

but with this progression I survive

Homebound til Further Notice

there's a symptom that angers me

it has me as dizzy as a hamster that flipped up inside the wheel

dizzyness has been a quite mystery

I've tried scopolamine patches, compound cream, seabands

but nothing sends the halting demands

lately it's been gone for a while

I say it's for the reason I've fallen

and my head adjusted

in all honesty, I never know when these spells come

they're so sudden

I try to stay homebound

for, the nausea has caused many embarrassments

so I'll stay homebound til further notice

'cause I never know when vertigo will strike again

FAmily

the best decision I've made was learning about my disease

my education increased

about the anatomy and about genetics

I'm more full of FA academics

5 years ago I wouldn't of been able to even say "Friedreich's Ataxia"

without a wave of shame drowning me like a tsunami

FA use to be esoteric

now I can even state the definition backwards

it has aided, my openness to the FA community

I say it was based on maturity

I don't feel much uncertainty

don't get me wrong, happiness comes hard but I have days where depression comes harder

I've learned it's more common than not

I have found people I relate with, finally

it's funny how the first 2 letters of family is FA

ABOUT THE AUTHOR

Yesenia Ramos is a creative, very imaginative, empathetic and committed person. She and her brother were diagnosed with Friedreichs Ataxia (a disease rare and incurable), at age 6 & 5. Ever since that young age, shes looked for a purpose. She's now 22 and her friend Ronald Salugao, who is a poet/music producer, introduced her to a coping mechanism so artistic; she fell in love with it so rapidly! Poetry has become her savior. This is her first book; where she shares her talent with words.

www.ingramcontent.com/pod-product-compliance
Lightning Source LLC
Chambersburg PA
CBHW030538220526
45463CB00007B/2882